Stop Overeating When what you Want is Sex

ISBN 978-1-5272-3948-7

Foreword

Are you tired of seeing other people having great sex and enjoying intimacy? Have you ever wondered why some people seem to effortlessly attract love and happiness, while you keep repeating the same pattern of being unfulfilled? Good! Then this is the book for you! This book will show you that you are more powerful than you know. You have the power to create the body you want and to get the sex and intimacy you want. It will help you to be in control of your feelings so that you can create the experiences you want and have all the love, confidence and energy you deserve.

Reading this book isn't enough; you must implement the tools that I give you and actively engage with the book. Eating when you are not hungry, choosing comfort foods and so-called 'treats' over healthy nutritious food, are signs that something is out of balance and you are using food to dissociate from uncomfortable feelings. At the root of most addictive behaviours is the need to numb out; this book will help you to stay present and move through the feelings without being overwhelmed by them. An absence of emotional nurturing and real connection creates a void that seeks to be filled, but it cannot be filled with food, however hard you try.

You have been pushed and pulled in all directions by the diet industry, as well as the media bombarding you with unrealistic ideals of beauty. It is time to stop punishing your body and psyche, and time to get your deepest needs for sex and intimacy met. When your needs are fulfilled in an authentic way, (not through food substitutes), the need to overeat will subside and you will begin to radiate a charisma that has eluded you all the years you have been trying to make your body look like someone else's.

The good news is that you can be rewired for optimal emotional health by learning to nurture yourself and heal the wounds that led to overeating in the first place. You will learn how to nourish yourself in the true sense of the word, and on every level, - emotional, spiritual and physical - all the aspects that make up what it means to be human and truly living. Sex and intimacy are as important as water and sunlight and you are entitled to as much sex as you want, in the way that you want and is most fulfilling for you.

You are not inadequate or broken, you are perfect! When you connect to that truth, it will support you in generating new behaviours - you will get a reality that reflects these beliefs, manifesting a body that you love and getting your most intimate needs met in a way that you never imagined.

So much has been written about self-love, yet after all the work of body positivity, very little has changed. Twenty-five years ago, we were being sold a beauty ideal by Supermodels and now their daughters are pacing the catwalk looking fashionably emaciated. You don't have to look like a model to be sexy! It is time to stop chasing after unrealistic ideals and come into alignment with your own beauty. It is time to stop denying your needs; you don't have to put your life on hold. Start claiming the happiness and fulfilment that are your birthright!

I share my knowledge and techniques with you in this book. This isn't a diet book, in fact it is the opposite of a diet book, however it would be unrealistic to expect to get healthy without making some adjustments to the food you eat. I give you the tools to make those adjustments easier. But don't let this book be a book that you read but don't actually implement the exercises. Please make sure that you put my advice into practice and you will marvel at the results.

Contents

INTRODUCTION

My earliest memories are of being comforted with food. Whether it was my Mother putting me in front of the television with a bag of sweets, or my Grandmother consoling me for being excluded from games with my siblings with a piece of cake, food became inextricably linked with love from an early age. It was set in stone deep in my psyche that food was my friend. I learned that food, particularly sugar, was a quick and readily available drug that could alter my emotional state - picked last for the netball team, told off by a teacher, snubbed as the boy that I liked sent the Valentine card to someone else - no problem, I found comfort in a bag of chocolate buttons or a Chelsea bun from the cake shop on the way home from school.

Being a very active child, I didn't gain weight, but at 13, the onset of puberty changed that: I developed curves seemingly overnight. I had stretch marks and hated my body. I began dieting and this was the start of a 15-year obsession with food and weight. I was either on a punishing diet depriving myself, or bingeing. With every diet I tried, I would gain more weight after losing it. I lived in a body that I hated, and after years of abuse, I finally reached a weight of 60 lbs over what is recommended for my height and was a size 18.

I knew I couldn't subject my body and soul to another gruelling diet, and I came across two books that helped me look at the psychological and emotional components that inform binge eating; The Only Diet There Is, by Sondra Ray and You Can Heal Your Life by Louise Hay. Reading these books began my journey to freedom and I will share the knowledge and techniques with you in this book.

All the time I was dieting, my body was my enemy. I learned to cut off from my feelings and deny my needs, which meant that for me sex was shameful, and I never truly got my need for intimacy met.

As I studied the books and implemented the tools and exercises suggested, the weight began to melt away and I began to be a healthier size, I was learning to love my body and started to wear sexy clothes instead of constantly hiding in baggy things. I was no longer staying in my room with a bag of comfort food but started going out to parties and night clubs; a whole new world of fun was opening up for me.

It was during this time in a sweaty basement club in Clerkenwell, that I met someone who would have the most profound effect on my life. Thomas was a beautiful Scandinavian guy with a body carved out of stone and staggeringly handsome. After a few dates, he invited me back to his place and to say that we had sex would be a massive disservice to him; it was more like a soul-changing, deep spiritual experience. What he didn't know about sex could probably be written on the back of a postage stamp.

After two days together, I called in sick at work and we continued our amazing love fest. After two weeks of dating and the most energetic sex, the weight was whittling away. I arranged to meet a girlfriend for lunch, as I walked into the restaurant and sat down beside her, she exclaimed, "Oh my God, you have been fucked gorgeous!"

That dear reader, is where I will get you. You picked up this book for a reason, you know that you are not having the best sex that you could be having, maybe you aren't having sex or intimacy at all - a sex anorexic. All that is about to change. Sex is a need as crucial as breathing and water. Without sex and intimacy, people become grumpy and disconnected. The French even have a term for it - mal baiser - maybe you had the misfortune to work with someone like this, they are cranky and short-tempered. If only they let themselves have fabulous sex, what a joy they would be to be around.

When was the last time you had really great sex? I'm talking about headboard thumping, hair messing, slam-you-into-the-middle-of-next-week sex? Or maybe there was no headboard in sight because you couldn't wait until you got through the door and had to rip each other's clothes off in the lift. Sex is natural and you deserve to be having it as often as you like and as much as you like.

Sex produces endorphins and chemicals better than any work out, it is great for the skin, increasing blood flow and circulation, giving you a glow that can't be bought in a jar. Stop spending money on expensive beauty products and let your real beauty emerge by having fulfilling sex.

It is time to stop disowning and disconnecting from your sexuality. We live in a society that makes us feel inadequate so that we buy things and the diet industry is a constantly growing billion dollar one. Diets do not work. Go into any bookstore and you will see a hundred books on dieting and losing weight. If one of them worked, there would be no need for the other ninety-nine. In recent years, there has been a flux in the market of books addressing the emotional aspect of overeating, and I would like to say that this would be the key for you to stop demoralising diets, but it isn't enough. Pick up any women's magazine, and I bet it will contain something of the following: an article on how to love and embrace your body as it is, an excerpt from the latest best-selling diet book and a recipe for cupcakes. No wonder we are confused!

Don't let this book be a book that gets relegated to your book shelf along with all the other things you tried. You will have to actively engage with the book and do the exercises. You have been shamed and manipulated for too long, it is time to stand in your power. I will give you tools and techniques that will help you to change negative states and feelings that no longer serve you, to help you immediately and permanently. I will guide you towards getting the love and intimacy that you want and deserve in a healthy way that includes boundaries. When you get your intimate needs met, you will no longer feel the need to self-medicate with food and chemical-laden sugary drinks. Until we find true nourishment and nourish ourselves, at the deepest soul level, we will always feel hungry, no matter what we eat. The Buddhists refer to 'hungry ghosts' that wander the earth, looking for love, so hungry for connection, but like bottomless pits, they never feel fulfilled. We, as a society, are over-consuming on empty food, junk food, fast food, and these are not really food, they are food-like substances, a weak imitation of food with little or no nutrition, leaving us craving more.

The same thing is happening with sex and love. Television, media, and the obsession with celebrity, means that we look at famous couples having spectacular sex and we feel inadequate and are always seeking to fill the gap. It is a never-ending downward spiral.

There is a way sanity can be restored. Self-worth is the healing balm that you can apply, and this book will help you to cultivate a deep and lasting sense of self-worth and self-love. So much has been written about self-love, but few have a real understanding of what true self-love is. This book will help you get to a feeling of profound and unshakeable self-love.

Chapter 1
Stop numbing out your feelings

Beth came to see me because she was a size 20 and at 5′, she was starting to feel as wide as she was tall. Working as a buyer for a big department store meant that she had to look good, and despite having beautiful hair and skin, she was finding it hard to feel good and project the image that she wanted. She couldn't find the clothes that she liked in her size and, like a lot of my clients, was resorting to dark and loose-fitting outfits. She noticed that more and more she wasn't feeling confident going into meetings, no matter how well she did her hair and makeup. She wanted to release the weight, but had tried so many times, only to discard a diet in the early stages or have some success but quickly regain all her weight. She said I was her last-ditch attempt.

Beth was a single mother of two small girls and saw herself first and foremost as a 'Single Mum'. Beth had an abusive childhood with a cruel and narcissistic Mother who neglected her and whose focus was on getting male attention and having affairs. Trembling with tears, Beth recounted a story of how at the age of 11, her mother left her on a park bench outside a flat whilst she went and spent the afternoon having sex with her lover. Beth's crushingly low self-worth meant that she ended up in an abusive marriage. She overate to deal with the loneliness and unhappiness and when she finally mustered the courage to leave and take her two daughters, her weight spiralled out of control. She thought that starting a new life would mean that she could also begin a new diet, but she was either working long hours and turning to take-aways at work, or when she was at home, wanting to be the ideal mother to her kids, so was constantly baking.

In our sessions, we unravelled what was really going on for Beth. On the surface, she was a successful career woman with two healthy, happy kids, but she knew that she was sabotaging her career by not presenting herself in the way that she wanted. She told me that her main aim in life was to be a great mother and always be there for her daughters in a way that her mother was incapable of. She felt that being a 'Mother' meant looking a certain way and she cited Ma Larkin from The Darling Buds of May - cosy and homely. After going deeper with a hypnosis session, Beth realised that she equated being slim and attractive with being like her mother - promiscuous and out all the time with a string of different lovers. We worked on getting Beth to see that it was safe to have an attractive body and that she could have boundaries in place and be in control, she would not be out every night neglecting her kids. Once Beth started feeling in control of her own sexuality, the weight fell off dramatically.

Beth was able to pinpoint the beliefs that were making her overeat and keeping her in a large body. She also came to see the irony, that in making herself big in body, she was keeping herself small in life and not really reaching her highest potential in her career. It is possible for you to get to the reason you have been holding on to weight and not letting yourself have an attractive body and the fulfilling sex that you want. We live in a world that titillates sex, makes it something "naughty" and women who enjoy sex are often demonised. We only have to look at the way things play out in the media, such as when David Beckham allegedly had an affair with a personal assistant, she was witch-hunted, branded a slut, home-wrecker and he emerged squeaky clean, eternally portrayed as a 'Family Man'. It is not a level playing field for men and women when it comes to enjoying sex.

I grew up in a small town and it was drummed into me by parents, sisters and women in the community that don't, whatever you do, get the reputation of being slutty. I soon realised that it didn't take much for girls in that town to be thought of as slutty. Meanwhile the boys were enjoying carnal pleasures without any slurs on their reputation.

I want you to do the following exercise to help you to release all the negative programming around sex. Firstly, let me make it absolutely clear that you are never to send this letter. Now get a pen and plenty of paper, or if you prefer to type then you can do that.

I want you to write a letter to your parents or your primary caregivers stating all the messages that they gave you around sex. So, it maybe something like "sex is dirty", "sex is shameful" or "sex is something that has to be kept secret". Really give yourself permission to get everything out, and remember this letter will never be sent, so no feelings will be hurt. Make sure that you have plenty of time and personal space to write this letter and don't hold back. Think right back to childhood and not just teenage years; often children are shamed for touching themselves or being inquisitive about body parts. Begin the letter "Dear (insert Mum, Dad or name), the messages you gave me around sex were…" Keep writing even when you think you are done, there is always more, so dig deep even if it is uncomfortable. If you feel yourself getting angry or crying, that is the goal. Remember that this is safe, no one but you is going to see it.

Now that you clearly see the messages you received and the belief systems you bought into, you can begin to unplug from that consciousness. It can be painful to look at this, but pain is a wonderful catalyst for change and feelings buried deep never die. By feeling them instead of numbing them, you will connect to a new way of being in the world. The only way out is through. The emotional body creates the physical body or, as Dr Bruce Lipton so succinctly puts it: "Your biography becomes your biology." What you are feeling determines your weight and body. You grew up with negative messages around sex and probably experienced shame which led you to cut off from your most authentic needs. You then put in place certain habits and patterns to manage the shame.

Often an addiction is just a way to manage pain and overwhelming emotions. Overeating is a subconscious pattern that tries to protect you but know this - a pattern and set of behaviours can be changed, it is not your identity, you can shift effectively from the pattern and get unstuck. When you act compulsively, you have no choice, but try and see the pattern for what it is, a set of beliefs. Just as easily you learnt them, you can unlearn them and learn more empowering beliefs, the truth of who you are, powerful and in complete control of your body and who you choose to have sex with.

The reason you overeat is that you have been living your life based upon a feeling of incompleteness that you have been trying to fill. Now that you are learning to connect to more supportive beliefs, they will generate new behaviours and you will get a reality that reflects those beliefs - living in a healthy body that you love and getting your intimate needs met in a way that you never imagined.

Chapter 2
Talk yourself into it

Like a lot of my clients, Fiona came to me wanting to resolve her issues around overeating and weight gain but there were other more pressing issues going on beneath the surface. An only child of a critical and abusive mother, she had a fierce Inner Critic that seemed to echo the pernicious put-downs that her mother dealt out on a daily basis.

"My Dad wasn't around much, I think he took refuge at work, but when he was, he wasn't very supportive or encouraging either. I remember him saying he didn't know why he paid for me to go to private school when it was obvious that I would never be a high achiever."

Fiona told me she was never academic or clever, yet she had built a successful career in advertising, having started out as a secretary. She felt that her vicious Inner Critic was sabotaging her work as she would often let other people take credit for her ideas, and she could easily give praise to others but was unable to give it to herself or celebrate her achievements. Like many people with poor self-image, Fiona always entered into inappropriate relationships, usually with men that were unavailable, and always with men that belittled and undermined her.

Fiona regressed to speaking like a scared little girl when she recounted how her mother would pick on her, rattling off a list of her personality flaws always ending with the terrible words, "No one will ever love you". Fiona had been in a heightened state of terror and that statement pitched deep into her subconscious mind, embedded itself there and became the basis for all her thoughts about herself, her body, and what she felt she deserved in life.

I worked with Fiona on silencing her Inner Critic and diminishing the power that it wielded over her. She was very conscientious in implementing the techniques that I taught her, and soon began to see the results showing up as a dramatic change in the quality of men that she dated, and taking care of herself to a level that allowed the sabotaging eating behaviours to subside and a real beauty and radiance to emerge.

I am going to give you a tool that will powerfully deal with your Inner Critic and negative self-talk, but you must implement it. You must always be vigilant and use this tool, never being lax. I call this technique, "Going Momma Bear". If you have ever visited a country where there are wild bears, a tour guide will give you advice on what to do should you encounter a bear. Anyone will tell you that if you have the misfortune to cross the path of a female bear with cubs, it is a highly dangerous situation, as she will protect her cubs fiercely from any threat or even a perceived threat. This is how fierce you have to be with that inner voice that criticises you.

I want you to step outside of yourself for a moment, and think about the things you say to yourself, "You stupid cow", "You look huge in those jeans", etc - would you honestly say these to someone else, or to your children if you have them? I am willing to bet that if someone did say that to your child, you would leap in to stop them.

Why do you think it is acceptable to speak to yourself in that way? It isn't. Never. Ever. It's non-negotiable, no matter how bad a day you are having, the second that Inner Critic starts, you get Momma Bear on it, you stop it in its tracks straightaway, not letting it get one little bit of momentum, defending your psyche, your soul and your self-esteem. Nobody deserves this punishment and as of this moment, you are never allowing it into your head and your life again. Your success in getting the intimacy and the body you want depends on this. Put this into practice like your life depends on it, because it does. If you are vigilant, this technique will work like a charm in your life.

One of the main modalities that I use in my work with clients is hypnosis. It isn't a mind-bending, mystical thing, it is simply guiding you into a very relaxed state, a state that you enter very naturally when you 'drift off', like when you are driving and suddenly reach your destination and wonder where the last 20 minutes went. It is known as the 'delta' or 'theta state' and this is the state that small children are in most of the time, which is why they are so susceptible to anything we say. Young children accept it as the truth, hence Fiona taking in her mother's words, that no one would ever love her, and her accepting that suggestion as real.

In just the way you were negatively programmed, it is possible to re-programme your subconscious mind. Again, the subconscious mind isn't a mysterious thing. There are two parts of your mind power; the conscious mind which is the logical planning part, and the subconscious mind which records habits and where all memories and experiences are stored. Imagine a big department store that has a manager - that is the conscious mind - giving directions. The subconscious mind is the staff, it takes and accepts the instructions given. You have been subtly hypnotised your whole life! For instance, every time you see an advert with a model looking a certain way that is deemed beautiful that doesn't match up with how you look, you register it as you being inadequate, or falling short in some way.

You don't need to go through your life being at the mercy of what somebody else tells you is beautiful, usually because they are trying to sell something. You can get back in the driving seat, and that is what I help people to do on a daily basis, by taking control of what they say to their subconscious mind. If you programme your subconscious mind in the right way, it will take you where you want to be. The mind will do everything to make reality match the belief and statement embedded in the subconscious mind.

So far in your life you have had a programming and conditioning that limits you and is full of self-doubt, but all that is about to change for you. Now that we have removed the vicious inner critic and the limiting beliefs, we can replace them with more supportive ones.

Negative self-talk was keeping you from having the body and the sex you want. Your thoughts create your body, and now that you are changing those thoughts, what shows up in your life will change. You will have a new reality that includes magnetising people and relationships to you that are in line with your new high self-regard. Faulty thinking was the only thing separating you from all that you want and deserve, and that is what created the blocks that kept you in a body that you didn't want.

The reason that many affirmations don't work is that you haven't effectively removed the deep self-doubt and programming. If you consistently practice the Momma Bear technique, it will dissolve a lifetime of limitations and get you to a point where your mind is like a fresh blank canvas, ready for you to put in the thoughts and beliefs that support you, so that you are restructuring your identity in the present moment, unencumbered by the past.

If you don't remove the deep programmes, it is like spraying air freshener near a damp wall; it will go some way to masking it, but the smell is always there underneath. This is how many people are going about trying to address their low self-esteem and issues around food and body image, putting on a red lipstick and saying "I love my curves". It isn't enough! I would love to say that it was, I really wish it was that simple, but years on from all the advertising campaigns about loving your body, nothing has changed and eating disorders and body image distress are on the rise.

You must bring in the subconscious mind, and when the conscious mind and the subconscious mind work together as a team instead of being in conflict, it will start to feel like you have a powerful ally. I am going to give you an exercise to do; it is simple, all that is required is that you are in a quiet place and will be uninterrupted. Get really comfortable, either lying down or sitting back in a comfortable chair, take a really deep breath from the pit of your belly and exhale. Do this three times and, as you exhale, let all your thoughts and stresses go, just drifting away.

Now focus on your feet and clench them then relax them; now clench your calves and relax; then squeeze the thigh muscles and relax; now focusing your attention on your buttocks, clench them and release. Put your awareness onto your stomach, pull the muscles in and release. Now scrunch up your shoulder really tight as if you are going through a narrow space, then relax. Now clench your fists really tight, so tight that you can feel your nails digging into the palms of your hands, then let go. Clench your jaw really tight, then relax. Screw up your cheeks and eyes, hold for a few seconds, then let go.

You are now relaxed, every cell of your body bathed in a lovely warm sensation, and every breath that you take makes you deeper and more relaxed. Just allow yourself to spiral down even deeper into the deepest relaxed state, where now we are accessing the subconscious mind. The subconscious mind only ever takes on what it is told and what it thinks is best. In the past it took in information that it was given that may not have been the most helpful and supportive. You are ready to do something different now, and welcome in a new life and a new way of being. In this deeply relaxed state, I want you to think back to a time in your life, a time when you felt on top of the world.

Now for some, this may be a time when you won a prize at school, or it can be a recent memory. If you don't have one, then conjure up that feeling in you now, because it is your natural state to feel good, you have just forgotten how. Now make that feeling even stronger, turn up the brightness, the volume, and with your right index finger, rub the back of your left hand just below the knuckles of your little finger and the next finger. The feeling of being happy becomes really strong now and know that you can access the feeling any time in the future by rubbing that spot. In this lovely relaxed state of a deep knowing and connection with your worthiness, mentally repeat the following statement: "I am perfect", then inwardly affirm it over and over until you are possessed by it.

Chapter 3

Smile with your vagina

Helen booked in to see me to address her lack of confidence. A very pretty girl with flawless skin and long honey-brown hair that was nearly always tied back in a severe bun, it soon became obvious to me that Helen didn't lack confidence, she lacked charisma. She was very clear that one of her goals was to get a boyfriend, yet despite working in a mainly male environment of a large IT company, she struggled to meet men. While I partially agreed with her that it may not be a good idea to mix business and personal relationships, she said that they were always going out after work for drinks and social activities, so there were plenty of opportunities for her to meet someone. I noticed that Helen always wore trousers, usually a dark suit.

When I asked her about this and suggested moving out of her comfort zone with her wardrobe, she told me, "When I go shopping and look at skirts and dresses, they always look a bit tarty." Then Helen opened up about the strict convent school she attended.

"At an all-girls' school, we didn't have a lot of contact with boys and we were discouraged from mixing with them after school. I remember one day I put on some bright pink lip gloss as I was leaving school, I was only 13 and I thought it looked great. As I left the school grounds, a nun saw me, she grabbed me by the arm, marched me back into the toilets and made me scrub it off at the sink. I was so humiliated, I think that is when I began to shut down any interest in the way I looked or in being feminine. I just channelled everything into school work and being sporty, pretending that I wasn't interested in fashion and thought it was shallow."

Helen didn't just shut down her interest in expressing herself through clothes and fashion, she completely cut off her sexuality and became disconnected from it. She told me that she met a lot of men in her active social life but, "They seem to look right through me, I never get noticed, and the men that I know through work call me a Ladette."

It was clear to me that we needed to reconnect Helen with her feminine essence that had been drummed out of her. After the sessions with me, she started to wear skirts and seemed less serious, not just in her dress sense and how she wore her hair, but in her whole demeanour. Helen really was committed to making the change and did the exercises I gave her diligently. I knew she would be successful. Like a lot of my clients, she kept in touch and six months after our sessions, she told me that she had started dating the owner of a restaurant that she had been going to for years, but he had never noticed her before. All of a sudden, she was showing up in the world in the most wonderful way.

I have seen many celebrities in real life, they don't always possess the most amazing physical attributes or beauty, but what they all have in common is a presence, a charisma that transcends physical appearance. The good news is that this charisma can be developed by anyone! The following exercise will help you radiate a confidence that is irresistible. I call it, "Smile with your vagina" and, instead of smiling with your mouth - which is lovely and you can do as well - you will be giving off an energy from the area at the back of your stomach referred to as the solar plexus.

Stand with your feet hip width apart, take a deep breath and gently shrug your shoulders up and down and really begin to feel relaxed in your body. Now bend your knees and use your hands to pull up the energy from beneath your feet to your stomach, take a moment to feel the warm energy there as you visualise diamonds at the top of your legs and your inner thighs and that pure diamond light entering through the vagina and into the solar plexus. Now put your arms out in front of you, make two fists then pull your fists up to your ears. Take a deep breath in and as you exhale, bring your hands down to your stomach. Again, let your hands rest over your stomach and stay there, really feeling the heat that is starting to generate there.

Now visualise a beautiful black cherry, really notice its shiny skin and imagine your tongue running over it, going into every dimple, every crevice. As you lick the cherry, feel it press against your lips and also connect to the tingling sensation in your solar plexus. Now standing straight, feet hip width apart, rotate your pelvis in a clockwise direction, round and round feeling the energy between your legs becoming stronger. You are now activating your powerful sexual energy and can radiate this vitality out into the world whenever you choose, and anyone you meet will experience a wonderful sensation from the charisma that you emit. Whenever you are in a situation where you would usually smile at someone that you find attractive, just visualise that erotic black cherry and it will bring up that feeling in your solar plexus. You will be smiling and radiating out from that area, you will be fully anchored in feeling sexy.

You can do this any time you choose, even if you are just walking down the street or entering a room, but be warned, this exercise is powerful, and once you become connected to your sexual core, the results will be nothing short of miraculous.

Chapter 4

What you are holding on to, is what's holding you back

When Sally first came to see me, she sat down and said, "I am sick of being the victim, I want to break the pattern." Whilst I agreed that this was a great intention, I told her that a better term might be to 'Heal the pattern' and she agreed with me. Of all my clients, she seemed one of the most willing to look at her part in recreating and repeating destructive patterns and relationships in her life, particularly around food and not valuing herself. The youngest of five children, she had what she described as a rough upbringing, where money and resources were in short supply and it was 'dog eat dog'. After her parents divorced when she was four years old, her father moved to another town, remarried and started another family.

Contact with him was irregular until she became an adult. Sally's mother worked two jobs and was constantly stressed and explosive, frequently having histrionic and violent outbursts. Her brother and sisters acted out this abuse, and were bullying and violent, and she witnessed brutal beatings. Her memory of her childhood was of "constantly feeling like I was treading on eggshells". Sally did what a lot of children in abusive family systems do, she developed a compensatory behaviour in order to survive, she became very quiet and knew that she mustn't 'rock the boat' or it would set her mother off.

Being constantly on edge and hyper vigilant, meant that Sally was often distracted and couldn't concentrate at school, so despite being bright, she fell behind. One of the few things she liked about school was the free school dinners as she was given so little food at home. Sally experienced severe neglect and she remembers looking through bins for food and as a teenager going to the houses of friends and stealing food from the kitchen cupboards.

Extreme neglect of this nature really impacts a child's sense of self-worth and Sally told me that she remembers thinking, "If my own mother and relatives don't think that I am worthy of food to sustain me, then I can't be worth anything." Sally hated her body and began doing things in an attempt to change it, she hated her breasts and developed round shoulders and bad posture. She couldn't remember a time after the age of 16 when she wasn't on a diet and said she felt happiest when her body was 'small and skinny' but every diet was followed by a period of bingeing and gaining weight, long periods in isolation, locked in her room with carrier bags full of crisps, biscuits, cake and chocolate.

She realised that she also felt good when she was fatter and wearing baggy clothes, "I felt invisible and non-threatening, like people would leave me alone and not pick on me." Sally's life had been characterised by going from one abusive relationship to another, and she made the observation that even if they didn't start out dysfunctional, she would soon make them that way, starting arguments and provoking fights. For someone like Sally, this is what love looked like.

If someone was abusive to her or put her down, she thought "This feels right". She told me that all her partners had been critical of her body, and one partner was constantly pointing out diet and weight loss products and bought her anti-cellulite cream for her birthday. She told me she was a size 10 at the time! She also had an abusive relationship for four years with someone that didn't want to have sex with her, he would either make excuses or sometimes initiate sex but not get an erection.

This further compounded her feelings of body hatred. Sally was very clear that she had a lot of anger in her and held on to a lot of resentment towards her family and ex-partners. She said that she was fed up of dating the same type of man over and over again, fed up of doing low paid jobs and of not letting herself have the health, sex and fulfilment that she knew deep down she deserved. Once we healed the pattern and removed the memories that were stored in her on a cellular level, Sally felt free and began to move forward with her life in a way that hadn't been possible for her when she was trapped in victimhood.

Sally deserved to find peace, but the choices she kept making only reinforced her poor self-image. There is a fable of a wise man seated in front of a large audience of his students and followers. He tells a joke, and everybody laughs, he then repeats the same joke word for word and people laugh less. He then tells exactly the same joke and punchline again, but this time, nobody laughs.

He then says to his students, "Isn't it interesting that you can only laugh at the same joke twice, yet we tell the same sad story over and over again, and cry every time?" Every time we tell the story of how bad it was, and recount the bad treatment we suffered, it becomes more and more hardwired into our energetic system and we become identified with the pain. I showed Sally that she was able to create a new identity and self-image based on the truth of who she was.

One of the best techniques I know to powerfully reboot the energetic system is E.F.T. (Emotional Freedom Technique) or you may have heard it referred to as Tapping. Known as being like acupuncture without the needles, it can transform an unwanted emotional state instantly. After attending an excellent training in E.F.T. with Peter Delves, I learnt more from the creator of the method, Gary Craig. He very generously gives lots of free information on the website, www.emofree.com. I will outline the basics of how to do a round of tapping but do go to the website for further information as this tool is transformational.

Take the index finger of your right hand and the next finger and rub the area a few inches below the collar bone where you would place a rosette or badge, thinking of the unwanted state or feeling, it can be a word like "angry" or a phrase such as "I'm not deserving". Keep rubbing that spot, and say "Even though I am feeling I'm not deserving, I deeply and profoundly love and accept myself", then take the fingers and tap the area where the eyebrows begin at the top of the nose, saying, "This feeling of not deserving" then repeat the words tapping the outside edge of the eye, under the eyes, then the area between the top lip and nose, then below the bottom lip, then under the arms near the bra strap, all the while repeating the phrase.

Then raise your eyes sharply up towards the sky and swiftly down to the floor, hum two bars of "Happy Birthday to you!" and rub each arm from shoulder to wrist as if you are rubbing off some dust. Now repeat the whole sequence and move into some positive statements, start with "Even though I wasn't feeling deserving, I deeply love and accept myself" then with each area you tap, say something positive like "I am choosing to feel something else" or "Letting this feeling go now". Do a few rounds of the tapping and you will notice the unwanted feeling subside.

There is no need to keep reliving past wounds, holding on to resentments that will continue to draw to you to the very circumstances you are trying to escape. Forgiveness is a crucial component to you moving on and creating the life you want and deserve. Forgiveness doesn't mean that you are making what the person did OK, it is saying "I am no longer willing to carry around the burden of resentment". Being angry with someone is like drinking poison and expecting your abuser to die.

They are not affected by your vigilant anger and are going about their lives blissfully unaffected, it is you that carries the weight of the anger and bitterness. Give yourself the gift of letting it go. Every minute you are angry, you have lost 60 seconds of happiness; don't prolong the suffering any longer, your life is too precious. It is possible to train your mind to be stronger than your emotions. One of the best ways I came across to really implement forgiveness and clear all grudges that we have long held, is a Hawaiian Prayer named Ho'oponopono which was devised by Dr Hew Len, who was working in a psychiatric hospital in Hawaii that was high security, where the patients were so dangerous and violent that they had to be strongly medicated and shackled.

As Dr Hew Len read through patients' records, he noticed what he was feeling and began 'clearing' what he felt. The term 'clearing' means to take all the programming, thoughts and beliefs, and erase them. As he looked at the patients' notes, he recited the following Prayer: "I love you, I'm sorry, please forgive me, thank you." As he cleared, he felt the patients getting well. Within months, the patients' mental health improved, medication was decreased, there was no need for shackles or straight-jackets, and many were released into the community. Ho'oponopono is about taking responsibility for your life and clearing any thoughts and beliefs that no longer serve you.

Some of my clients initially say, "Why should I say sorry?" and have difficulty using the word 'sorry' when they are not the ones that did something bad. But this is not saying sorry and admitting fault, it is petitioning the Divine, so that energy is cleared and it is possible to move forward untainted by the stored memories that are painful and difficult. I recommend that you use this prayer frequently and particularly when you want to neutralise challenging situations with potentially toxic people.

I find that as well as doing a spiritual and emotional cleaning and clearing on a regular basis, it is also a good idea to do a physical cleanse. One of the best ways to do this would be to have colonic irrigation to remove all the built-up debris and toxins in the gut, as extra weight and bloating could be faeces blocked in your colon. The colon is the last part of the digestive system and its role is to eliminate waste. If the toxic waste is accumulated, it can have serious implications on your health both physically and mentally, making you feel heavy and sluggish.

The poisons pollute your bloodstream and impair the proper absorption of nutrients. If you don't like the thought of having a tube put up your bum, or the cost is prohibitive, then I know a way to cleanse the gut with a herbal laxative, that is as effective as a colonic but doesn't remove the good gut flora. Buy a packet of Potter's Herbals Cleansing Herb Tea, which you can purchase at any good health food store or online. Put a level tablespoon of the herbs in a big mug and fill with boiling water, allow to steep for 30 minutes.

The best time to drink it is around 9 pm and don't eat anything after drinking it that night. When it is fully steeped, drink the whole mugful; it doesn't taste nice, but the benefits are worth it. Please be warned not to take this if you will be travelling around a lot the next day or in long meetings, because you will need easy access to a toilet as you will have a lot of eliminations, and they will be strong. Please do not do this at all if you are pregnant. The day after this you will feel much lighter and I recommend that you begin to cultivate the healthy and helpful bacteria in your gut by taking a good probiotic or Kefir. You can purchase probiotics in tablet and liquid form, but avoid the commercial ones that contain sugar.

Now that you are cleaning and clearing the unhelpful programmes, it is important to be vigilant about what you put in your system. As the body is 85% water, I recommend that you not only drink good quality water but also infuse the water with good energy by writing words on the bottle. A Japanese scientist, Doctor Emoto, conducted an experiment with water in which he wrote different words on bottles of water, some negative such as 'hate' and some positive such as 'love' and 'joy'.

After freezing the water, he examined it under a microscope and the water imprinted with the positive words showed up in beautiful shapes and forms of crystals and snowflakes. The water that had been imprinted with negative statements appeared squiggly and gnarly, discoloured and ugly. You can actually buy stickers to put on a bottle, but I just use a makeup crayon to write words. Write whatever you wish to embody the most, 'love' or 'beauty', or maybe what you most wanted to receive as a child but were never told, such as 'clever' or 'capable'. You are now wiring these qualities into your system and as you alter the frequency of your body, you will be vibrating at the frequency of your desire: love and fulfilment.

Please implement the techniques I have included in this Chapter on a regular basis and you will notice the benefits. In closing this Chapter, I would like you to spend a few minutes repeating the following statement: "I now lovingly release everything that no longer serves me."

Chapter 5

You Matter!

The spiritual teacher and writer, Eckhart Tolle, says that a story backed by a powerful emotion becomes a pain body, and on my first meeting with Mike, despite his big grin and firm handshake, I could sense his pain strongly. "I want to get rid of this" he blurted out as he rubbed the big belly that was bulging over the belt of his trousers, but as we talked about his life and what had brought him to seek help with his overeating, he was candid in opening up about a sex addiction that had been active in his life for a long time, and that had come very close to sabotaging his marriage and other areas of his life.

With an absent father and a mother who put him into care at the age of seven, Mike had serious abandonment issues. His story was that he wasn't wanted in the world and not good enough and the emotion behind this was one of deep sadness, leading to his pain body. "Between the ages of seven and sixteen, I was in and out of care homes and foster homes. Some kids that were fostered got adopted by the foster parents, but that never happened to me. I always thought that if I had been cuter, nicer, then I would have been taken in and loved by someone."

Mike had a deeply held belief that he was unlovable and behaved in a way that was consistent with that belief, being a people-pleaser, always seeking approval and validation. The inner landscape and whole psyche of an addict is one of lack and scarcity, they are like bottomless pits and never feel full or satisfied. As a child, to cope with his chaotic childhood, Mike adopted a strategy of making people like him so that they wouldn't reject him. "I would always do extra chores in the care homes to ingratiate myself with the carers and it was the same when I was placed in a foster home, I didn't let my guard down for a second, always making sure that I wasn't demanding or much trouble."

This continued into his early adult life. "I learned magic tricks to impress girls at parties and it never failed, I even got the nickname Action Man because I got so many girls, but deep down I felt that I always had to be doing something to earn someone's love and attention." Mike began to realise that in his unrelenting pursuit of love and sex, he was actually abandoning himself and bringing about the thing that he feared the most, and not just bringing it about but hardwiring it to his very core.

Mike told me that his sexual conquests felt empty, and like all addicts, he would seek more excitement and admitted that he was taking more and more risks, sometimes not practicing safe sex by using a condom, or revealing too much personal information that could lead to his wife finding out. Mike was in a punishing cycle of self-abuse and self-hatred. After getting a job as a salesman aged 17, Mike forged an impressive career in Sales and became an international sales director of a big company, but it was clear to me that Mike could never feel his achievements.

There is a term: Imposter Syndrome, where people feel that they shouldn't really be in the place of success that they are. Over the years, I have heard many clients say that they only got into a prestigious University because there was a drive to admit more people from state schools or that they only won an award because the other competitors were weak that year. Imposter Syndrome just means an inability to own your talents and accomplishments. It was becoming more and more clear to me that this was the work that Mike had to do in order to become whole.

Mike was addicted to approval and was always seeking it, but in our work together, he came to realise that he was very rarely getting his needs met, although one area in which he felt that he could reward himself was food. He often ate out in expensive restaurants and when on the road with his job would order a Chinese takeaway for four people and eat the whole thing.

In one of our sessions he admitted that he had bought a McDonald's takeaway and eaten it on the way to my office.

Mike soon realised that what he termed 'treats' weren't real treats and that the true definition of a treat was to take care of his body and take the time to eat healthy food. He knew that every time he was 'grabbing something on the run', even if it seemed like something delicious or indulgent, it was reinforcing his belief that he wasn't deserving of time and attention. Mike was able to slowly introduce habits and behaviours that enabled him to get his needs met and see them as valid rather than negating them in order to make people like him. Mike loved a saying that I quoted, "You can't be everybody's cup of tea, otherwise you would be a mug" and joked that he would get a tattoo of those words.

I don't know if Mike ever did get that tattoo, but what I do know is that as he began to see that he mattered in the world, and that his value wasn't dependent on him doing anything or earning it, his chronic people-pleasing subsided and his need to over-indulge in food and unfulfilling sex stopped.

Mike experienced a painful wound as a child and was always operating from that wound. He made the decision that he was unlovable and not worth anything, he could not bear to be with his feelings and was constantly trying to numb them out. People in the grip of addictions think that their feelings are too painful to feel, that they will overwhelm them and eventually kill them, but feeling is healing and denying is dying - a slow death where you learn to mask your emotions, develop a false self and over-compensate for feelings of inadequacy with fake bravado. Let me define what real confidence is.

It is not to be confused with those loud, brash arrogant people. True confidence is possessing a deeply held belief that you are deserving of life's riches, that you have as much right to them as anyone else and that you are worthy. Your needs are relevant, and you matter. There comes a point where you have to realise that your worth is a given and you don't have to earn it.

You don't have to work hard or manipulate people into loving you. One of the biggest buzz terms in the last few years has been 'Self-Love', and books and articles will tell you to practice self-care and have beauty treatments. Whilst I am the first person to rave about a great lipstick and think that whoever invented the bubble bath should receive a Knighthood, those things only scratch the surface when it comes to self-love and healing.

The problem is that you are told to do something else to take you away from the feeling of wanting to overeat or whatever the unwanted behaviour is, but this is just another way of distracting yourself and not being present. Where the real power lies for you is to be present with the feelings and know that it is OK and you will move through them. You don't always have to be up, you can love and accept yourself when you are feeling down, it is OK to be there for as long as you need to be there.

Of course, you want to put an expiry date on feeling bad, and you can get over the bump in the road, but it is important to acknowledge where you are and not negate those feelings. Mike was always trying to distract himself from his feelings and the original pain with overeating and empty sexual conquests, but the further he got away from himself, the lonelier and more disconnected he felt. Mike began to really feel his achievements and hold an experience by practising something that I shared with him - gratitude. Mike was always wanting more, but the practice of gratitude helped him to 'line the pit' and really feel full.

Gratitude will work wonders in your life, it gives us the ability to stop comparing ourselves with others and begin to feel our own blessings. Gratitude doesn't have to be just for the big things like a house or car (although do be grateful for these things!). It can be for the smallest of things; turning on a tap and getting water, a sip of a cup of tea, a child laughing on a train. When we look for things to be grateful for, more things appear.

I would like you to keep a daily gratitude journal and write everything that you are grateful for, big and small. Even on bad days, remember to express gratitude for the things that can be taken for granted - eyes to see, legs to walk, ears to hear music. Be grateful in every moment and watch your world transform. One of the biggest ways we signal to ourselves that we don't matter is in how we feed and nurture ourselves. Clients will often tell me that fresh fruit and vegetables are too expensive, but they will happily spend on gifts for others or on ready meals because they don't have enough time.

Be conscious of the time you give yourself to eat. From this moment on, I don't want you to ever eat while you are walking or rushing around, checking emails, opening letters or other tasks. When you eat, you are communing with the soul and this is a sacred time. I once heard some priceless advice, "Whenever you eat, imagine you are in front of your future in-laws", in other words, always take the time to use a knife and fork, eat slowly, savouring the food. So many people bolt down their food, not really tasting or enjoying it or allowing it to digest properly. Even if it is a small thing like an apple, take the time to really smell and taste it. You will begin to feel more satisfied and you are sending yourself the message that your needs matter as much as if you were entertaining and feeding the most esteemed guest.

People with a poor sense of deserving find it hard to receive compliments, in fact they are not good at receiving at all, they will bat away a compliment because feeling good and getting attention in a positive way feels uncomfortable and they can't wait to get back to the state of feeling shitty because feeling shitty is what they are used to. You may struggle with accepting a compliment or maybe even doubt that the person means it sincerely.

If you want to really begin to get the sex that you want with partners who value and respect you, then you must learn to receive a compliment and hold it. No matter how much you are tempted to make a self-effacing joke or belittle the value of the compliment, don't. Say "Thank you" and breathe it in, let it sink deep into the core of your being. Find a quiet place and sit comfortably, take a few deep breaths and quiet your mind. Take a deep breath from the pit of your belly, then make the following statement: "I matter". Keep repeating until it feels comfortable. You can make this your mantra, and if you like you can even make it a tattoo!

Chapter 6

Coming out of Shame

Debbie had tried many different types of therapies to address her weight issues and chronic back pain, going on retreats, seeing different doctors and taking lots of different medications. Nothing seemed to work for her and although sometimes she had a degree of success with releasing the weight, the results were never long lasting, and she would always revert to what appeared to be her set point weight of 15 stone. At our initial meeting, Debbie repeated the same sentence a few times, "Something is missing".

Debbie told me that her early childhood was almost idyllic and laughed when she said, "there was even a pond with ducks in the middle of our village."

However, Debbie's parents were obsessed with image and presenting a united front to the world, but as Debbie got older, she realised that there were cracks in her parents' marriage. In an attempt to hold the marriage and family together, her mother became more and more preoccupied with making the home look good and entertaining.

"It seemed like Mum was only interested in her kids to the extent that we could make her look good, she loved to show off about our academic achievements, but in private she was cold and critical. I remember taking a cookie from a jar and she bellowed across the kitchen, "Little pickers wear bigger knickers.". My brother and sister thought it was funny, but I remember feeling humiliated.

Debbie described her home life as, "barren and joyless" but, as a teenager, she discovered that a way to get attention was to be promiscuous, and having sex with boys meant that she was getting some semblance of love and attention. At the age of 15, drunk at a party, she ended up in a bedroom kissing a boy, three of his friends came into the room and they coerced her into having sex with all of them. She said that she felt a terrible sense of shame and didn't want to tell anyone, but word got around and a few days later a boy passed her on the school bus and shouted, "You big slut.".

"The general consensus seemed to be that because I was promiscuous, I would have sex with anyone, and nobody seemed concerned that it had happened against my will. I struggled to make sense of it all, but I wasn't emotionally mature enough and I ended up internalising all the feelings of shame and self-loathing." Debbie continued to be promiscuous and had no boundaries around her body, when she moved to a big city at 18, she thought she could be anonymous, and no-one would judge her but the deep feelings of shame stayed with her. Partying, drinking to excess, eating erratically and self-medicating with junk food, she began gaining a lot of weight. She would occasionally attempt to diet but would quickly regain all the weight and more.

"I just hated the idea of dieting or even healthy eating in any way, it would drive me mad when my friends talked about calories all the time and bought diet food, and I know it was because it reminded me of my Mum and the importance she put on appearance, so overeating felt like a big two fingers to a world that was telling me I had to look a certain way."

In our sessions, Debbie confessed that the promiscuous sex she was having was unfulfilling and she used sex as a tool to get people to like her and was always focused on pleasing the person she was having sex with, never considering her own needs and often agreeing to things that she didn't really want to do. She realised that the overeating served two purposes - to numb out her feelings of ever-present shame, and to create a big body, showing up in the world as what she called "big and scary" so that no-one would abuse her or take advantage of her again. However, she knew deep down that this wasn't working and in some ways she was perpetuating the abuse and making it more active within her.

She said that whenever she would lose the weight, she felt, "Cold and exposed, without my protection." In our sessions, we worked with putting the shame where it belonged, with the boys who had violated her, and that she didn't need to embody it and constantly continue the abuse by not valuing and neglecting her health and body. She could see that the body she was creating wasn't working for her, and in fact it disempowered her, she was tired from carrying around the extra weight and living her life as a shame-based person, which had informed every area of her life. She made excuses not to apply for jobs she wanted and didn't take part in hobbies and activities that she was interested in.

As Debbie moved out of the feelings of debilitating shame, she began to be less concerned about what people thought of her and started to honour her body, knowing that it was safe to have a slim body and that all that had been missing for her were effective boundaries, and she now had the self-worth to put these boundaries into place. She didn't have to agree to anything she didn't want to do, and she loved "The Two Cs"; consent and condoms, which had to be present whenever she was having sex with someone.

If, like Debbie, you are overeating and creating a bigger body as a way of sticking up two fingers to the world, then please stop, nobody is noticing, the only person you are harming is yourself! In every moment, you are making a choice about what you put into your body and food is either healing or hurting you. You have suffered enough punishment, don't perpetuate it with the use of foods that make you feel terrible.

In my work as an Eating Disorders Counsellor and Hypnotherapist, I saw clients present with many different issues, but an alarmingly high percentage had one thing in common, they were sexually abused or violated. People that were sexually abused often take on the shame of the abuse as if they were the perpetrator, they feel tainted and flawed and embark on a myriad of ways to punish themselves, not least of which is abusing their bodies with food and denying themselves any real soul nourishment.

When we feel flawed and defective, it is hard to be authentic, we feel that we have to cover up our true selves with an adapted self that we think is more acceptable. Coming from our wounds of toxic shame and isolation, we create a false persona and our real self becomes more and more removed, ashamed and disconnected. This book is about getting the sex you want, the amount and quality that is right for you, and that you feel comfortable with, without being burdened by societal judgement. People that didn't receive love in a healthy way and were put down or ignored, find it hard to receive love, so they create substitutes, or they will seek out partners that can't fulfil their needs, people that are rejecting and unavailable.

If you see a pattern in your life of pursuing people that can't meet your needs, don't think that you can change them, looking for love from these people is like going to the hardware store to buy milk, you will never get it. The relationship expert, Barbara De Angelis, says that if you take the five words that describe your childhood home that you grew up in, you will have your relationship described. I asked Debbie to describe her childhood home in five words, (You can also use terms such as "always treading on eggshells" or "looking for affection"), she used the words, 'cold, lonely, disapproving, shallow, empty'.

She was alarmed at how accurately that described most of her relationships, she often got together with men that were cold and shallow, incapable of giving her the love that she sought and not interested in satisfying her sexual needs. It is OK to ask for what you want. I have a friend, Jeff, who says that when going down on a woman, he writes each letter of the alphabet with his tongue and then the woman can say which letters are her favourite and hit the spot, and these are the letters he will use.

Unfortunately, not all men are this aware and ready to please a woman, but you can ask and you can tell whoever you choose to have sex with what you like and how you like it. It is possible to disentangle from the toxic and unsatisfying experiences of the past and create new neural pathways in your brain, you no longer have to hold on to painful baggage. It is safe for you to get love, sex and intimacy, and you can manifest your ideal body, regardless of what anybody else says is the right amount of sex or the right shape of body. No more punishing yourself or moulding yourself into something that is not right for you.

Debbie was creating pain in her body and the chronic back pain was a way to not feel painful emotions. When she brought her shame out into the light and stopped repressing her feelings, her back ache subsided and her health improved. Let me make the distinction between responsibility and blame, as I want you to see that you have responsibility for your life. A lot of people think that if they take the responsibility, it is saying that they created things in their past and are to blame for them.

You are not to blame, but from this moment on, you are absolutely responsible for how you feel and how you respond; nobody can make you feel anything, you have one hundred percent control over what you feel. The model and activist, Amber Rose, decided that she would reclaim the word Slut after receiving so much criticism and vitriol aimed at the way she dressed and the number of men she dated. Every year in Los Angeles, she organises a Slut Walk, where everyone can dress as sexily as they like.

She started the Slut Walk to support people that have been shamed and show them that you can come through it with dignity. She said that one young woman came up to her wearing a grey sweat-shirt and sweat-pants, and told her "This is what I was wearing when I was raped." If you think that creating a fatter body or wearing baggy clothes will protect you from being attacked or violated, you are wrong. Sexual attacks are about the misogyny that runs deep within our society and the only way we will ever change anything is to reclaim our bodies, our sexuality and say that we will wear what we want, have the sex that we want and have the body we want without fear of criticism.

You are an incredible human being that is so much more than the size you are, you no longer have to be in shame or hide your sexuality, and you don't have to disown and disconnect from your body. Women like Amber are shining the light on the double standards that exist in our world around men being applauded for sexual activity and women being shamed. Women hiding will do nothing to shift this attitude. However, what will halt it, is educating people that No is already a complete sentence, we don't ever have to justify or explain it. No means NO and consent must always be present.

I want to say something about the body positive movement where people are standing up to size discrimination and saying that they are proud to be a bigger size. Often the women at the forefront of these campaigns are very confident. I saw one of its most vocal protagonists, Amy Schumer, the writer and star of I Feel Pretty - a film about body confidence - being interviewed by Oprah Winfrey and she shared that she grew up with the most encouraging parents who made sure she knew how beautiful and clever she was and that she 'totally bought it'. That is wonderful for Amy, but sadly most of us didn't receive this sort of positive reinforcement.

I can remember reading a conversation between Meghan Markle and a journalist in which Meghan said that as a child, she didn't like the freckles on her face and her father told her that a face without freckles was like a night sky without stars. If only we had all received that kind of love and validation of who we are from our families. Instead we were criticised or made to feel wrong in some way and every time we are shamed, it goes deep into our neurological wiring.

After years of this wiring, it is hard to instantly love the way you look. This is called 'spiritual bypassing' and it means trying to escape and gloss over parts of you that you find painful to look at.

It is like trying to stop a train travelling at 80 miles per hour and suddenly making it go in the opposite direction. You must let the years of self-admonishment and crippling self-judgements fall away, find the trauma within you that started the cycle of self-punishment, and know that you can build new neural pathways in the brain. You can change the molecules by consistently cleansing and clearing your thoughts so that you are in the present moment, a clear space where you let go of your story and wounds and instead, connect with the truth of who you are, a beautiful soul.

When you reach point zero, or your home frequency, your authentic self begins to shine through, not a false self that you constructed to protect yourself. Your body is the physical form of your thoughts and you can change your thoughts and emotions and propel them into matter - creating the body you want.

One of the best ways to release old unwanted emotion and really be present in the moment is through breath work. I would like you to do the following exercise for the next 14 days, taking 20 minutes every day. It can be whatever time of day that suits you best, find a quiet place where you won't be interrupted, all phones and devices off or on silent. Lie down on your back with your legs straight or with your knees drawn up pointing to the ceiling, whichever is most comfortable for you.

Take a moment to really be in your body, settle into it, relax the jaw, shoulders that may be up near your ears, let them drop and take a nice deep breath from the pit of your belly and really feel the connection to your pelvis and that area, loosening up. Close your eyes. Now take a deep breath in through the mouth and out through the mouth. This may be different to some breathing and yoga techniques you have done where you breathe in through the nose, but this is the best way to really open up the pelvis where you hold a lot of tension.

Keep taking the breaths in and out through the mouth and remember, how when a puppy or baby breathes, their little bellies rise and then gently go down. This is what you are aiming for. So many people are shallow breathers, breathing from the chest, whereas these deep breaths will be a wonderful detox that will reboot your nervous system. As you continue to breathe deeply, noticing your belly rise, and let yourself be aware of the space an inch behind the bridge of your nose; now visualize and feel an opening for a few minutes.

Now visualise the colour pink and with each breath you take, send the pink light energy to every part of your body that you have ever disowned or disliked, sending love to those parts of your body that you have hated or neglected. Now let that pink light go to the base of the spine, let it go up every disc of the spine up to the back of the neck, then to the crown, down the front of the face to the throat. Breathe in this pink light, seeing every cell of your body as healthy and loved, as you breathe out, release all unwanted habits you have held in place.

Let the pink light go down below the belly button, now contract the muscles of your pelvic floor, as if you were having a pee and were stopping it mid-flow, now as you contract those muscles, breathe in and send that healing light wherever it needs to go. As you continue to breathe deeply, you are now opening up to receive all the good in the world that is ready to be bestowed upon you, and you are developing the wiring of honouring and celebrating your body, being conscious of your sexuality and only ever making choices from a place of good self-esteem and high self-worth. Mentally repeat the following words three times: "It is safe for me to show up and be who I am in the world."

Chapter 7

Chemicals: why you keep overeating

Tara sought my help to overcome her carbohydrate addiction, but it didn't take much delving to reveal that she was actually relying on a number of foods, drinks and stimulants to manage her moods. Tara didn't have any trauma in her childhood, but she told me that her parents always used food as a reward system. "If I helped my Mum with chores, she would take me to the corner shop where I could choose some sweets, and when I passed my driving test, I called my Mum and she said, "Oh great, I'll get a cake". I remember at school I would look at the clock all afternoon and long for the bell to ring so that I could get a can of Coke and a KitKat on the walk home."

She told me her teenage years were characterised by "doing silly diets" and laughed as she told me her friend had the great idea that smoking and drinking coffee made you lose weight. "I followed a seven-day diet from a magazine with my sister, at the end of the week we had each lost a few pounds, so we rewarded ourselves with a cream cake." She said that her weight and eating habits were "all over the place" but the one constant whether she was dieting or not, was sugar.

On discovering that wine gums and jelly babies had a low-fat content she would binge on them. Tara said that she always had mood swings and her work mates even gave her a mug stamped with the words, "Give me the coffee and no-one gets hurt". In our sessions, we looked at the not so funny side of her mood swings, she admitted that she once picked up her boyfriend's phone and smashed it against the wall in a fit of rage.

She was able to see a pattern in her life where she had always used carbs and sugar to regulate her moods. She would grab a Danish pastry and coffee on the way to work to "get me going".

By lunch-time she was ravenous and would buy a sandwich or wrap, when she got back to her desk it wasn't long before she experienced a dip in energy and around 3pm she would head to the break area for biscuits or go out and get a coffee and chocolate brownie. When she got home in the evening, she felt exhausted and too tired to cook, so she would put a frozen pizza in the oven or boil some pasta because it was quick and easy, later that evening she would crash out on the sofa to watch TV and eat cookies.

"I can never have just one or two, I eat the whole packet, I don't seem to have an off switch, or if I go out for dinner with friends, I will get home and make toast, even though I know I can't be hungry." Tara had a clear intention - to be free of the tyranny of this addiction and the mood swings.

Tara was not stupid by any standard, all that she lacked was critical knowledge about the way in which certain foods impact the body chemistry and inform binges, Once she was armed with that knowledge, she was able to take back control of her life and restore balance. In recent years, I have seen a flood of books about mindful eating and intuitive eating, but they are missing a vital piece of information, and that is how thus far your unhealthy eating habits have impacted your body chemistry and blood sugar. I know from personal experience when you are at the mercy of this chemical roller coaster, sitting down and asking, "Am I really hungry?" or "What am I feeling?" just won't cut it. Likewise, when people advise "Just don't have trigger foods in the house", you will swim the Thames at 2 o'clock in the morning to get the food you are craving and only that particular food; if it is Ben & Jerry's Chunky Monkey that you are craving, Häagen-Dazs won't do!

Refined sugars and refined carbohydrates were wreaking havoc with Tara's blood sugar and body chemistry. Sugar and wheat in their original form do not cause dramatic spikes in the bloodstream, in just the same way that cocoa leaves that grow in South America will not give a dramatic high, but give a very light buzz akin to drinking a weak cup of coffee. However, refine it and pare it down, and you have the drug cocaine, which if you take it, causes a powerful surge in your body or what we call a high.

It is the same with other drugs, such as heroin that derives from a poppy plant; when that plant is refined and pared down, it becomes a highly addictive substance known as heroin. Refined sugar and refined flour that form the basis of carbs like cakes, cookies, white bread and pastries light up the reward centre in the brain the same way that drugs do. There is nothing to buffer the hit they deliver, so it causes a rapid peak and dopamine is released, dopamine is the chemical that is produced in the part of the brain that is associated with reward.

Nature had to create a reward system in our bodies to make sure that we did it again, so that we would procreate, because sex felt good. In nature, there wasn't that much availability of food, so overflooding the system with dopamine didn't occur and in turn, a dramatic rise in blood sugar didn't occur either. However, today there is a constant availability of food and the modern, Western diet contains a lot of refined carbs and sugar and diabetes is on the increase. Your body requires blood sugar for energy, but it can't cope with an excess and will go into crisis.

When blood sugar level goes up, the brain signals to your pancreas to send insulin to the bloodstream. Insulin will help your body to either turn that sugar into immediate energy or store it, thereby regulating blood sugar levels. The body can't cope with the onslaught of blood sugar that the modern diet produces, and insulin levels become too high, and then blocks the hormone, leptin. Leptin is a crucial hormone that tells you to stop eating, letting you know that you are satiated, don't continue to eat, but go out and work or hunt.

This is why you no longer get the signal to stop eating, because you no longer have that inbuilt system that nature devised. Your high sugar and high refined carbs, which act like sugar, have produced too much insulin in your body. So, you are on a roller coaster of getting blood sugar highs, then crashing, then needing more and more to get some sort of hit or energy surge, and never getting the stop signal. The good news is that leptin can be restored, and your blood sugar can become stable so that you can get off the roller coaster and its associated mood swings.

You are beginning to see that refined sugar and carbs are as addictive as drugs, the only difference is that you can buy them on any High Street and they are completely legal! Not only is the addiction just legal, but it is openly encouraged! Think of the many adverts, such as the one for Pringles - "Once you pop, you can't stop" that make fun of your inability to get the stop signal. If you have been in the grip of a sugar and carb addiction like Tara, you will know that it isn't a lot of fun. You can find balance and regain sanity.

This isn't a diet book, it is the opposite of a diet book, but it would be unrealistic of me to expect you to stop overeating without making some changes to help you have the freedom that you deserve. One of the changes is to cut back and reduce refined sugar and refined carbs. I hear you cry, "Oh no, not another protein diet, how does this differ from all the other low carb diets like Atkins and Keto?" The difference is that those diets are unsustainable, there is no flexibility in your food choices and makes it impossible to live your life free from obsessing about food, not to mention that they give you bad breath and constipation.

You don't want to forego the cake at your friend's wedding or not be able to have a dessert after a meal in a restaurant if you want one. What you do want is to stop putting your body into a high chemical response by spiking your blood sugar, so don't go for long periods without eating and then, like Tara, go for the big hit of a food with a high glycaemic load like a chocolate brownie or a pizza, and especially not a glass of white wine.

As I said before, this is not a diet book, if you do want to look further into the subject of nutrition and how to have less refined carbs in your diet, then I recommend the books and research of Dr Mark Hyman. I don't advocate that you remove white carbs completely, but I do recommend you aim to make them 15% of your diet; 25% of your diet protein and 60% good fats. Good fats include avocados, cheese, particularly goat's and sheep's cheese, organic eggs that are high in omega-3 fatty acids, dark chocolate, oily fish, grass-fed butter (the cows are not fed on grains) extra virgin oil, coconut oil, Udo's oil, nuts and nut butter, chia seeds and plain full fat yoghurt that is not sweetened.

This book is about you enjoying food more, not less, and not depriving yourself in any way. Once you start to introduce more real foods into your life and have less fake food or 'Frankenfoods', you will really connect with the joy and pleasure of eating.

You can cut loose from the crazy chemical swings and roundabouts brought on by a high sugar and carb lifestyle, but I have to mention that the chemicals produced by toxic emotions are just as bad and far more damaging than any e-numbers found in food. Your body has an inbuilt fight or flight mechanism; if there is a perceived threat, your body floods with adrenaline and cortisol so that you can either fight the animal that is attacking you or flee from the situation.

Except in modern life it isn't a bear attacking us, it may be a boss making demands, or having to multitask.

Your body thinks that it is in a stress situation and you may be going into a famine, so it stores fat, and this fat usually gets stored around the middle. It isn't just stress that produces cortisol, but our own toxic feelings of anger and rage. There are lots of ways to calm your nervous system; deep breathing, meditation and my favourite – gratitude. Don't wait until you lose something to appreciate it, whether that is your health, a relationship or certain privileges you have - appreciate them today. There is also another option to fight or flight and that is to freeze. In nature it may have kept us alive if we played dead and didn't move, but the modern-day freeze response is hiding, withdrawing and wishing things were different. You don't have to freeze, you can be moving and showing up in life.

You have seen how chemicals have had an effect on your life and now it's time to realise that you have nature's pharmacy at your disposal. One of the best ways to produce feel-good and wellbeing chemicals like serotonin in your body is through exercise. Dr. Andrew Weil, a holistic health doctor, says that the number one antidote to depression is exercise. What is the best exercise for you? The one you are most likely to do. There is no need to join expensive gyms unless you like them. Walking is one of the best exercises ever and is free. Exercise should be fun and one of the best ways to have fun is to dance.

The movement of dance creates a powerful vortex of energy that really elevates your mood. Find a dance class near you and sign up. Zumba is fun. I highly recommend that you check out 'Soul Fire Dance Party' by Josette Tkacik, which is an online dance course. Josette is a Zumba teacher, she is great fun and you can do it in your own home, although I do think that you can't beat the fun and connection of going along to a class with other people.

Which brings me to the subject of connection. One of the best ways to release serotonin in the body is to get a hug from someone, preferably for 20 seconds or longer. Lots of cultures hug as an everyday occurrence, so make it a common practice for you, ask for a hug and see your world open up as you start to feel more connected.

Saving the best 'til last, nothing beats sex as a form of exercise. Great sex opens blocked energy channels in the body and improves blood circulation. It causes the production of heat in the body which improves the metabolism. When your body goes into the sexual response of excitement and arousal, serotonin is released, the heart rate increases, giving you a full cardiovascular workout, dopamine is released, and your sympathetic nervous system makes norepinephrine stimulate the brain, making the genitals more sensitive to pleasure.

At orgasm, oxytocin peaks as muscles rhythmically contract and built up tension is released. You don't have to have a partner to enjoy these benefits and in fact you should make pleasuring yourself a necessity whether you have other people to have sex with or not. I recommend that you stimulate your clitoris to the point of orgasm as often as you can during the day instead of seeking out the fleeting hit that is provided by carbs and sugar. It is much more satisfying to climax, easy to do and will give you a long-lasting glow.

Make time to visit a sex boutique, I love Coco de Mer in Covent Garden, London, I do realise it is a bit pricey and you might want to visit one that fits your budget, but whichever one you choose, this is your time and I want you to buy some beautiful underwear that makes you feel sexy. The model Elle McPherson said that she could always tell the British models when they were getting changed for fashion shows because they had grey underwear with bits of elastic sticking out!

It doesn't matter whether anyone is going to see it or not, beautiful underwear shouldn't be saved for best, it should be worn every day, celebrating and honouring your vagina and breasts. Your sexuality has been hijacked by the pornography industry and sexy lingerie is often associated with porn magazines or lads' mags, but it doesn't have to be. This is for you and about you reawakening your sexuality and getting as much sexual pleasure as you want.

As well as buying underwear I suggest that you treat yourself to some sex toys although you can just as easily stimulate your clitoris with your fingers or a shower head. Having a powerful orgasm isn't just about the genitals, it is about having a full body orgasm and feeling the excitement rise through your whole body, sending a tingling sensation everywhere, even the toes, as pleasure and arousal heightens and experience that wonderful oxytocin rush. It's better than a sugar rush any day!

Chapter 8

Stop deifying chocolate

A lot of my clients make the first call to me because something happens that makes them realise they are not living their optimal lives and they are ready to look at how they can do things differently. For Charlotte, it was holidaying in Paris and being obsessed with finding a particular café - Angelina's on the Rue de Rivoli - that she had heard served the best hot chocolate in the world. "I was so excited as I made my pilgrimage there, and it didn't disappoint, it was like liquid chocolate in a cup, and as I sat sipping it and watching the chic Parisiennes with their lap dogs and Chanel handbags, everything seemed right with the world."

It may seem harmless to visit a café in Paris that has been recommended, but Charlotte was going out of her way to go there most days of her holiday. "I knew on some level that it was crazy when there were so many amazing things to do and see in Paris, but I rationalised my behaviour by saying that this was the real Paris I was getting a snapshot of, not some tourist place near the Eiffel Tower, but deep down I knew that my obsession with chocolate was out of hand and on the plane home, I vowed I would get help."

Tryptophan is a chemical found in chocolate that causes the release of the feel-good hormone, serotonin in the brain, which explains Charlotte's blissed-out feeling in the café in Paris. It became evident to me that Charlotte had relied on chocolate to access this blissed-out state from a young age.

"Both my parents worked shifts and my Dad did a lot of the things like picking me up from school and making our evening meal. He would always have a bar of chocolate for me. There was a point where I wasn't very popular at school and two of my friends that I had always spent time with started doing things without me.

"No matter what I did, I felt like a misfit, but getting into Dad's car at the end of the school day felt like stepping into a portal of love and safety and as I munched on the chocolate bar or chocolate buttons that he had bought me, all my cares seemed to fade away. My parents worked hard to provide a stable home for us, but they weren't good at showing affection, I don't remember being hugged very much. They both demonstrated love through food, we never talked about things in our family, and even when I had period pain, my Mum would bring me a hot water bottle and a bar of chocolate.

"Things changed when I went to sixth form college. I got a new set of friends and I came out of my shell a bit, but I was never one of the pretty, popular girls, and boys didn't ask me out. I ended up having sex with a male friend and it morphed into him being my boyfriend, but the sex was awful, and I couldn't wait for it to be over. Without fail, after seeing him, I would go to a shop and buy chocolate to cheer myself up. I was doing OK academically but didn't seem to excel at anything and I sensed my parents were disappointed with me. In my late teens and early twenties, I slept with both men and women, I really didn't have a preference and remember thinking, "God, I can't even get this right, I can't be completely gay or straight."

'One of my happiest relationships was with Anna, who opened my eyes to a whole new way of living. She loved making healthy food and knew so much about nutrition. She had done a massage course and studied essential oils. We would go to the market and buy fresh fruits, vegetables, herbs and spices, it was so sensual. Sex was amazing and during my time with Anna, I felt more alive than ever before. This was the first time in my life when I wasn't preoccupied with chocolate. The weight fell off me and I had newly-found cheekbones. The penny should have dropped that it wasn't really chocolate that I wanted and there were lots of other ways that I could get pleasure, but when I broke up with

Anna, it coincided with starting work at a big PR company, it was a high-pressure environment and I reverted to old habits.

"My boss was a harridan, and in the way that some people smoke to cope with stress and anxiety, I turned to the chocolate that I kept in my desk drawer. The girls that worked there were effortlessly cool, they all seemed to live near the Portobello Road and have boyfriends that were DJs. They were nice enough to me, but I always felt like an outsider. There was a tradition of bringing a cake into the office when it was your birthday and, on my birthday, I bought a big expensive chocolate cake from Choccywoccydoodah. Everybody loved it and warmed to me more after that.

"It only confirmed my deepest held belief - that chocolate was the best way of bonding. There were often drinks and parties after work, but, more often than not, I would prefer to go home and watch TV or read, usually picking up some indulgent chocolate dessert on the way home. Sometimes I would go out with my workmates and we would get chatted up by men, but if they ever asked for my number or to see me again, I declined, thinking they were out of my league, so why bother. I remember at the office Christmas party that was held in a really swanky bar, one of the gay guys that I worked with said, in front of everyone, "Oh if you don't get a boyfriend soon Charlotte, you'll end up on the shelf, and with those hips, it had better be a wide shelf." I laughed, but when I got home, I burst into tears and had a hot chocolate and a packet of M&M's."

Charlotte knew that she was attributing chocolate with magical qualities that it didn't have, and she knew that there were other ways to bond with people and that chocolate wasn't the only way. Charlotte had a taste of what life was like without chocolate, being slim and healthy and getting her intimate needs met but her low self-worth meant that she didn't fully receive the experience and value herself enough to make it a way of life. How much you value yourself will determine the level of high-quality food and high-quality sex you will allow into your life. Charlotte had opportunities to go and have fun, but she turned them down. She had the chance to date quality men, but she refused them.

She knew about and could afford healthy fruit and vegetables but eschewed them in favour of convenience foods and chocolates. Real chocolate, with 90% cocoa solids, meaning that 90% of the weight comes from it, tastes pretty awful - it is only after the addition of fats and lots of sugar, that it becomes palatable. As well as containing Tryptophan, chocolate also contains Theobromine, a chemical that has a similar effect to coffee, it's a mild stimulant that produces feelings of well-being. Charlotte started to see chocolate for what it really was, cheap waxy crap with drugs added to it. It didn't have magic mystical qualities, and as for it being better than sex, Charlotte had experienced fantastic sex and agreed that chocolate didn't come anywhere near being as satisfying as that.

If you say that chocolate is better than sex, you have been having sex with the wrong people! We have seen so many adverts for chocolate where as a woman seductively puts chocolate in her mouth, she reaches a state that is close to Nirvana, we have been subtly hypnotised into believing that chocolate is some erotic experience, but now the dehypnotising begins as you start to break the spell that chocolate manufacturers and the advertising industry have had over you. Having chocolate occasionally is OK, and as I said in the previous chapter, a good quality dark chocolate is actually good for you and contains antioxidants.

People go to horse races a few times a year and have a bet on a horse to win, they are not gamblers, and they don't think about gambling until the next time they go. In the same way, you will be able to have chocolate occasionally if you feel like it or if someone has served a chocolate dessert, and not think about it until the next time you have some. If you have been eating a lot of chocolate like Charlotte, breaking free of the compulsion to eat it does have a physical component to it, because your blood sugar will dip. So, as a way of supporting you through the initial transition into your new way of being without chocolate as a constant crutch, I recommend that you take a supplement, Sucroguard, made by BioCare. It will help to stabilize your glucose levels and when you wake up every morning, drink a big mug of warm water with lemon juice squeezed into it. This will help adjust your taste buds, from the over sweet chemical products they have been used to.

My clients often complain that to eat healthily is expensive, yet they think nothing of buying chocolate from pricey chocolatiers. Start to go to markets and really spend time smelling the beautiful fruits on offer, nothing beats the smell and taste of a ripe mango or melon. Begin to connect with the pleasure that Mother Nature supplies generously, let yourself eat the colour of the rainbow in fresh fruit and vegetables. It isn't difficult to start introducing fruit and vegetables into your diet, and you are worth the effort! Every time you scrimp on your food budget or grab a snack that is cheap and convenient you are sending a powerful message to your subconscious that you aren't worth anything. Eventually we really are what we eat, you don't want to be cheap and tacky.

Charlotte not only had the experience of eating beautiful, healthy food when she was with Anna, but she also experienced the other sensual pleasures of massage and essential oils. I want you to start engaging all five of your senses, so that you become a fully-awakened sensual, sexual being. Our sense of smell is the quickest synaptic leap in the brain to our memories, and therefore smelling something triggers a feeling more strongly than anything else.

Essential oils vibrate at one of the highest frequency levels known, and the one with the maximum vibration is Rose Oil. The frequency of a healthy body ranges between 62 - 78 Hz (units of frequency). If you want to be vibrating at a high level at which you are attracting fantastic sex with amazing partners, then do everything that you can to raise your frequency. As well as eating high vibration fresh foods, I recommend that you incorporate essential oils into your life, in an oil burner or diffuser in your home, in the bath or shower and mixed with a carrier oil to massage your body.

Sound is another way to create a resonance in your body that connects you to a higher vibration. 432 Hz is believed to be the healing frequency. It is easy to find this music on the internet or listen to any music that you find uplifting.

This book is about how to stop overeating, and the irony is that overeaters often don't really taste food, as they are eating it quickly, not chewing it properly or savouring the tastes, textures and flavours. Eating blindfolded is one of the most sensual pleasures you could ever have. If you can be blindfolded while someone feeds you foods like strawberries, figs or grapes, then that is great, but you can do it on your own, or even just close your eyes as you taste a different variety of texture and flavours, maybe try chilli peppers with a dip that you like. Now that you are learning to engage the senses that you had forgotten about when you were turning to chocolate for a quick thrill, you are really seeing chocolate with new eyes; now every time you see it in a shop you think 'cheap, waxy crap'.

Whenever I hear people say that they are embarking on some diet, detox or boot-camp at the end of which they will look and feel amazing, it breaks my heart. You don't have to take time out of your life to begin feeling fantastic, you can start incorporating the steps I have outlined in this chapter now, without giving up your social life or foregoing invitations. Your life is for living, don't waste a moment of it in deprivation.

Charlotte realised that everything she wanted was already there and it was only her judgements that stopped her from having it. Thinking that the girls at work were cooler than her, making sweeping statements like, "they all seemed to live near the Portobello Road and have boyfriends that were DJs" that just weren't true, judging some men as being out of her league was, again, not true. Once Charlotte dropped the self-judgement that was causing her blocks, they were easily dismantled. She came to see that enjoying life and its sensual pleasures wasn't the preserve of rich people and that she wasn't less than anyone.

You have the right to fun, you have the right to be enjoying delicious food and even more delicious sex. Every morning when you wake up, open the curtains or raise the blinds, and with your arms open wide, make a clear statement to the universe "Bring it on!"

Chapter 9

Feeders

Arriving late for the appointment, Nadine slumped in the chair and announced, "I nearly didn't come today. I feel so guilty, my parents adored me, I have nothing to complain about", and that was the first clue of how Nadine felt overly responsible for other people's feelings. Nadine's parents were small children during the Second World War. Even after the war, there was still rationing, so as soon as rationing was over, their families loved to buy cheese, cream, butter and sweets whenever they could.

"My mum seemed to have this attitude of 'eat it today, you might not have it tomorrow', even though we were quite wealthy, and my Dad had a really stable job. All my school friends loved coming to my house; my Mum liked baking and things that were reserved for special occasions for most people, were an everyday occurrence in our home, Mum made cakes, muffins and biscuits, nothing was ever shop bought. Family dinners always looked like we were expecting lots of guests, not just a meal for our family of four. There was usually creamy mashed potatoes made with lots of butter and Mum would be upset if there was any left in the bowl. As a teenager, I very rarely left the house without Mum putting a snack in my bag or making me eat a sandwich, saying "You don't know when you will be eating next."

"I hated sports at school and always tried to get out of doing it. I was part of the arty crowd and it didn't bother me that I was starting to get chubby, I loved wearing combat trousers and Doc Martens. All that changed when I discovered boys and clubbing. I would put dresses in my bag and tell my parents I was going to study at my best friend's house. We would get into clubs and dance the night away; I started to lose weight and get lots of attention; I loved the feeling, and started skipping meals, throwing away the packed lunches Mum made me. All through drama school I was very slim, but then I met my husband. He was such a feeder; he loved cooking and would prepare elaborate meals with different sauces, and was always surprising me with flowers and chocolates."

Nadine went on to describe a happy marriage, but the reason she had come to see me was that as a professional singer, she wanted to look the best that she could, but whenever she dieted, her husband and mother would make her feel guilty if she didn't eat the indulgent food they prepared. "I work as a backing singer quite a lot, and often the artists don't want backing singers to look better than them, so it isn't a problem. But I want to do more of my own material, I want to look the best I can, I don't want to be in the background all the time." Nadine had no problem eating healthily and being disciplined, it was only when around other people that her resolve weakened.

"My Mum will say "but I made this cake especially because I knew you were visiting" and my husband says I'm no fun if I don't want to go for a pizza. All it takes is for friends to say, "Oh, go on" and I will have a glass of wine or dessert that I don't really want. Even when I hired a Personal Trainer and started to look great, I would undo all the hard work by eating the trifles and puddings my husband would leave in the fridge for me." Nadine knew that she was sacrificing her success by putting people's happiness first, but I was able to demonstrate to her that armed with the right techniques, she could stand her ground with the most persuasive of feeders.

You are not responsible for other people's happiness, when people try to force food or drink on you, don't take it personally, often they have their own issues around food that they are acting out. If you are in a social setting, it is OK to give an excuse, such as you have an allergy, or you are driving, and you don't want to drink alcohol, but only with people you don't know that well. With friends, family and partners, you are going to have to put firm boundaries into place, and in the same way that you don't have to have sex if you don't want it, you do not have to explain why you don't want to eat something.

Remember, NO is already a complete sentence. Feeders can come up with more and more manipulative ways to coerce you into eating against your will. If it is a close friend or relative, visualise a rose gold coloured bubble around you, their best attempts do not get through to you and just bounce back. Do not get drawn into a conversation, repeat NO THANK YOU and change the subject.

Nadine became a successful solo singer and looked every inch the part of the sexy, slinky Diva. Don't let anyone come between you and your dreams!

Close your eyes and take a few deep breaths, then repeat the following affirmation 10 times: "Nothing is more important than my health and happiness."

Chapter 10
Connection

Stella told me that she had always felt disconnected, not wanted, and unwelcome. "My Mum fell pregnant with me when she was 41, my two brothers were teenagers and although nobody said the exact words, it was always obvious that I wasn't a wanted child and I seemed to be a burden. I knew from the way that other parents behaved towards their kids that Mum and Dad were neglectful, but I just got on with it". Stella seemed quite stoical as she recounted the appalling level of neglect in her childhood. "If I ever had after school activities, my family would have had their meal by the time I got home, and Mum would leave food between two small plates on top of a saucepan of water for me to heat up. I never got treats, and once my parents even forgot my birthday!"

Stella didn't have nice clothes like the other girls at school, but got along by playing the class clown. "I had this incredible ability to make people laugh and would do impersonations of the teachers". Although it served her well, she admitted that throughout her whole life, she had felt as though she had to work really hard to make people like and accept her, and this extended to her sex life. "My first big relationship was with Jamie, a drop-dead gorgeous, but penniless, musician, I paid for everything.

"At first, the sex was really good, I felt so lucky that this super handsome, super charismatic man was interested in me. As time passed, I lost respect for him, I just didn't feel sexy in any way, but I didn't want to break up with him. I thought it was better to have someone than be on my own, so I stayed with him, going through the motions of having sex to please him. I would go to his concerts and look at all the gorgeous girls in the front row and wonder why he was with me, I totally lost myself." It was during this time that Stella's unhealthy habits started.

"As a kid, one of the ways I would escape the horrible reality of my home life was to go for long walks with our dog, I would get to the furthest away field that I possibly could and sit listening to music through my earphones while I ate a big bag of Haribos. At the end of my relationship with Jamie, I turned to food when I was miserable, Nachos with melted cheese and sour cream on top, and gummy bears, anything to try and blot out my sorrows."

Stella seemed to have enough self-esteem to get out of the relationship, but she embarked on a strict diet. "It was a bit depressing having a small tin of minestrone soup for lunch and not being able to go to the pub after work, but I stuck to it, and after a few months it paid off and I could borrow the clothes of my flatmates who had always been much skinnier than me. I went to a party hoping Jamie might be there and I could really piss him off with how great I looked, but I met Max that night, an incredibly funny, insanely-sexy stand-up comedian.

I noticed that Stella used similar words again, "I couldn't believe he was interested in me" and I could see her very poor self-image reappearing. "Dating Max was so much fun, normal rules didn't seem to apply. We would be in a restaurant and he would pull me into the bathroom to have sex, once we were at a big dinner party and he passed me a note that said, "I want to fuck you."

I asked Stella if she was happy during this time and she replied as quick as a flash, "Not really, I was wracked with insecurities, I was so jealous, I would go through his pockets, scrutinising receipts, looking for evidence of other relationships. I went through his phone bill checking numbers and I noticed that one call lasted 45 minutes. When I called the number, it was his bank". I asked Stella to connect with what Max liked and found attractive about her. "I gave him a lot of support I suppose, and helped him write his comedy material; I got an incredible buzz when I would hear my jokes on the radio the next day."

Stella displayed typical co-dependent tendencies - always supporting her partners in the pursuit of their careers to the detriment of her own needs. She admitted that she wanted to go on a comedy writing course but could never afford it. When we looked at ways that she could save up to pay for the course, there were lots of things she was wasting money on, such as a gym membership that she hardly ever used. Stella came to see the ways in which she didn't value herself enough to bring her talents and gifts to the world, and how she used food to check out from her dissatisfaction with her life. In our sessions, Stella was able to connect with her vision, and she did take the comedy writing course. Once she stopped living through others, she created a life that she didn't want to escape from with overeating.

People think that they are addicted to food and are powerless to break away from the compulsion to overeat, but I don't think it is the binge food that they want. In an experiment conducted in the late 70's, Psychologist Bruce Alexander built a 'Rat Park', a large living environment for 16-20 rats of both sexes, with food, toys to play with, wheels to run on and plenty of space for mating. In another experiment, rats in small cages were forced to consume a solution containing morphine for 57 days. When they were moved to the Rat Park, they could choose between the morphine and ordinary water: they drank the plain water and had only minor signs of withdrawal. What does this tell you? Bruce Alexander believes that it is the living conditions and not the addictive property in substances that make an addict, and I entirely agree with him. Once people start to feel connected, and they align with their innermost desires, both sexually and creatively, their need to self-medicate with food subsides.

The following exercise is one of the most important that you will ever do, so mark out sometime that you won't be disturbed, and find a place to lie down or sit back comfortably.

Imagine that a big birthday party is being held for you. As you look around the venue, really take in everything that is going on; the decorations, the music, the aroma of the food and drink. There is a stage with a microphone, and one of your closest friends takes the microphone and makes a lovely tribute to you, saying how much they love you and making a long list of your incredible attributes. Next is a close family member, (you can make this a parent, grandparent, sibling or child). As they take the microphone and begin to extol all the beautiful qualities and personality traits that you possess, really receive the love, let it flood every cell of your body. As you look around the party at all the people who appreciate you, take a moment to let it sink in.

Whenever you are ready, open your eyes and take a deep breath. Now I would like you to write down everything that people said about you, make a list of all the qualities that they loved about you. This exercise bypasses your ego. If I had asked you to list your best qualities, chances are you would have found a way to diminish them or be modest, but by doing this process you see yourself through the eyes of others, and let all your lovable qualities come to the fore to be celebrated.

Many people, like Stella, compare themselves to others as if they are in some imaginary competition where they always come last, it is time to stop the comparing and judgements; comparison will rob you of joy. Stella could never quite believe or connect with the fact that her partners loved and desired her even when she was having fabulous sex. She couldn't let herself really feel the bliss of being wanted and sought after. Keep the list of all your amazing qualities close by, look at them frequently and know that you are loved.

Chapter 11

My opinion on self-love

The term self-love has been bandied about so much in recent years, and yet the definitions that are offered seem so far removed from what love really is. The true definition of self-love is wanting for others what you want for yourself and realising that you are not separate from the world. You are no less deserving than anyone on the planet. We live in a crazy world where people drive to a gym to exercise, we go on dating apps to meet someone but don't talk to the person sat next to us in a café.

Many years ago, in a village in Thailand, there was a temple with a statue of a beautiful golden Buddha. One day news reached the village that an army was about to invade, so the villagers gathered mud and stones to cover the golden Buddha in the hope that the army would see no value in it and pass by. It was an effective ploy and the army charged by the statue without noticing it. Years passed until one day a young monk was meditating near the statue and a chunk of stone fell off revealing the gold. Villagers came with picks and chipped away the stone revealing the golden statue.

In what way have you covered up your talents and hidden your beauty as self-preservation? You were born golden, knowing your intrinsic value and worth, now it is time to reconnect with that truth.

Please take the time to implement the tools and techniques I have included in this book and you will realign with the truth, knowing that you are loved and deserving of all good things.

I mentioned earlier in the book the 2 Cs, which must be present whenever you have sex with someone: Consent - don't ever agree to anything you don't want to do, not for any reason, there isn't a reason. Condoms - always make sure that you practice safe sex; if someone is having unprotected sex with you, they will be having unprotected sex with others. Self-love is honouring your body enough to protect it. I would like to add a third C and that is C for Cab, if you stay at someone's place and have sex and intimacy with them, they should want to know that you get home safely and in comfort. Now go forth and have fabulous sex!

Further reading/ references

You can heal your life, Louise Hay
Louisehay.com

The only diet there is, Sondra Ray
Sondraray.com

The biology of belief, Dr Bruce Lipton
Brucelipton.com

Peter Delves, delves.co.uk

Gary Craig, emofree.com

Zero limits, Dr Ihaleakala Hew Len and Dr Joe Vitale
zero-wise.com

The hidden messages in water, Dr Masuru Emoto
Thewellnessenterprise.com

The power of now, Eckhart Tolle
Eckharttolle.com

The choice for love, Barbara De Angelis
Barbaradeangelis.com

Food, what the heck should I eat? Dr Mark Hyman
Drhyman.com

Spontaneous happiness, Dr Andrew Weil
Drweil.com

Josette Tkacik
Josettetkacik.com

Bruce Alexander
Brucekalexander.com